THE LOVE DEN DIARIES
VOLUME 2 – HEY GIRL IT'S OK TO SWALLOW

Disclaimer: This book is for the exchange of information NOT for the diagnoses or treatment of any kind. This must be left to a licensed professional; Always see a qualified medical practitioner before making changes in your health and fitness practices.

Advice given in this book or in conjunction with **The Love Den Diaries** (ANY

VOLUME) is not to replace the advice given by a licensed professional nor be taken as a counseling or clinical relationship but only as suggestions. As the reader of this series or user of **The Love Den Diaries** website you bear full responsibility for your decisions and actions. External websites linked from **The Love Den Diaries** series of books and The **Love Den Diaries** website are for information and reference purposes only. We do not endorse any product, service or treatment.

As a user of **The Love Den Diaries** website or reader of **The Love Den Diaries** series you bear full responsibility for your decisions regarding these products, services and treatments.

Table Of Contents

Chapter 2 -The fellatio frame of mind

In this chapter we will discuss how to mentally and physically prepare to do the deed.

Chapter 3 - Do I really have to return the favor?

Are you one of those ladies that feel like just because he goes down on me, that doesn't mean I have to do the same? In this chapter we will discuss why many women feel this way as well as the "swallowing double standard"

Chapter 4 - Become a dick sucking diva

Tips and techniques to give him some of the most intense, mind blowing orgasms he has ever experienced in his life.

Chapter 5 - Getting your girl to go down

This chapter is for the fellas. Are you are having issues in your relationship because she won't "go down?" Learn EFFECTIVE ways to encourage her to give you oral pleasure.

Chapter 6 - Double the pleasure, double the fun

Learn how giving head can be a gratifying experience for BOTH partners.

Chapter 7 - Practice makes perfect

It's just like anything else. If you want to get good at it you have to put in some practice time, this chapter will teach you ways to "perfect the craft

Introduction

"Hell no! Don't even ASK me anything like that! I don't go down on men. Only sluts do that. You want me to do what? And swallow what? I've NEVER done that, I Swear!"

These are just a few of the phrases used by women who refuse to give their man a blow job. They are convinced that the entire male genital area is gross and therefore must be avoided at all cost when it comes to anything oral. Sadly enough these same women demand that a man not only go down on them but to give multiple comatose orgasms all while swallowing up every bit of the juices they excrete.

There are also the women who fall in the opposite of this category. They won't even let a man's face even come near their neither regions for fear that he will ask that the favor be returned, as he rightly should, and so they have given up that part of sex altogether. Well I'm here to tell you girl, you are missing out!

Then there are the ones who can suck the skin off of a dick but refuse to admit it to anyone. They even have the nerve to put down other women who talk about their own personal experiences on the subject.

And let's not forget the lady who WILL actually go down on her man but she also secretly hates doing it. The only reason she does it is because he wants it. He usually has to ask for it, or should I say beg for it. This usually results in her bobbing her head up and down like a robot on his member and forgetting every other part of his body. The end result is not a pleasurable experience for either party.

In this series of The Love Den Diaries Volume 2- Hey Girl It's Ok To Swallow we will cover issues such as:

- Why some women are experts at the "craft," "super heads" if you will, and some are rank amateurs.

- Getting a better understanding as to why some women even in this day and age still view giving head to a man as taboo.

- Tips for the beginners as well as some advanced moves for the seasoned veterans that will have his body exploding with pleasure.

- How to mentally and physically prepare to do the deed.

- The "swallowing" double standard.

- Exploring the possibility of giving a man oral sex that's gratifying for BOTH parties. As well as picking up on cues and body language that let you know you're definitely hitting his "hot spot."

- Learning how to effectively communicate with your partner to create a bond that will last long beyond the bedroom.

So with that being said ladies, I humbly ask you to loosen your jaws and your minds. And prepare to "blow" his socks off!

Chapter 1 - YUCK! I don't want to do that!

It's been around since the beginning of time. The English noun fellatio comes from fellātus, which in Latin is the past participle of the verb fellāre, meaning to suck. Wikipedia describes Deep-throating as an act in which a man's entire erect penis is inserted deep into the mouth of a partner, in such a way as to enter the receiving partner's throat.

The term was popularized by the 1972 film Deep Throat. It may be difficult for some people to perform, due to the requirement of suppressing the natural gag reflex.

I know you don't want to believe the fact that your mothers and grandmothers gave blow jobs, but they actually did. The only difference is back then was that it wasn't socially acceptable to practice such debauchery. A person could be banned from their families, church or religious circle. Or in some cases even be placed in jail for breaking the law. In short it was something that was done, but was not spoke about.

Depending on your age category, religion, culture, upbringing or personal experiences, giving a man a blow job is considered to be taboo even in this day and age. Many women have been conditioned to think that sucking dick is something filthy and bad. And that only sluts and whores do that.

I can remember growing up in a household where sex was rarely mentioned. And when it was it was basically a brief conversation of just keep your dress down and your legs closed. God forbid if the topic shifted to it being something pleasurable for two people in a committed relationship. Oh yes, I know some of you grew up with parents who didn't mind talking about the birds and the bees with their children. Even still I can just about guarantee the topic of oral was off limits. That is of course you were being told not to do it because you would be labeled a "loose woman." In most respectable households the mere thought of bringing up oral sex would cause your parents heads to implode!

I can count on one hand how many women I have encountered over the age of thirty who had parents that were completely open and honest when it comes to sex. The majority of young people learned most of what they knew (which was usually wrong) from older siblings and or friends.

This generation of sexually uneducated children led to girls believing all kinds of bizarre rumors about their body. They were told everything from they could get pregnant from heavy petting to sitting on a boy's lap. Also think back to when you were a teenager to how everyone treated the girl in the neighborhood who slept with all the boys. Every block had one of these "sluts," "loose women," "whores."

Remember how she was labeled and scorned not only by you and your friends, but your parents as well? You had to make sure at all costs that you were not labeled one of "those" kind of girls. Some women had to grow up in strict religious environments where a woman's modesty was her virtue. This is actually a good thing, but you can see where it could cause inhibitions about sex later on in life.

Sex itself is something in most religions that's reserved for marriage. However that's not the issue. The problem comes in when a child is first taught that they are doing something bad if they touch their own body in an erotic manner or masturbates. You remember the old wives tale that stated you will go blind if you jacked off? I'm here to tell you EVERYONE in the world would be using a white cane if that were the case. Some parents even pitched a fit when sex education finally made its way into the schools. Despite the fact that teen pregnancy and sexually transmitted diseases were sky rocketing.

It is this lack of education and strict upbringing that have many women still denying that they have ever sucked a man's dick. And when and if they do preform the act it's with the look of repulsion and shame on their face.

I can remember being on a social network and a young woman posted the question: "Why do men assume all women suck dick?" Let me state that this was young woman in her 20s. I patiently awaited the comments that poured in. They ALL said the same thing. "I DON'T SUCK DICK."

Now I don't believe for one minute that these women don't give head. What the thread did show me was the fact that even though these were younger women and that the year was 2011, there was still a stigma behind openly admitting such a thing. It showed me that they were ashamed to say they had sucked a man's dick, hence the reason behind me writing this book.

I have explained some of the reasons that the older generation still finds it taboo, now let's touch a bit on the subject of why younger women feel this way as well. Granted, we live in a society where sexual freedom runs ramped. As a matter of fact that's an understatement. I have noticed that a great majority of people who are screwing any and every one like they don't have a care in the world are also careless about using protection as well.

These are the same people that will tell you that they went to a party on the freak train last week, but complain about a STD scare the next. It's like going from one extreme to another. Either people are total stiffs when it comes to talking openly and freely about sex, or they are total freakazoids in every sense of the word. Can we get some balance people?

There are plenty of women bold enough not only to admit that they don't mind giving a blow job, they will admit to swallowing among other things as well. These same women will also outright ask a man that they barely know to suck his dick. So why is it that even some of the women in this group will still lie about it around other women when the topic arises? Is it for fear of being judged or ridiculed?

In my experience with speaking to this

generation of young women, bold or not, some of them are indeed ashamed but for different reasons.

Most of the younger generation of women who do in fact suck dick but wouldn't admit to doing so was because they were either sexually abused or made to do so as a child. And the pain and shame stays with them even as an adult.

Or they didn't know their own self-worth and were sucking dicks all willy nilly. Meaning they didn't have to be in a relationship with someone for them to perform oral sex on them. A guy didn't have to be special in any sense of the word, as long as he told them what they wanted to hear or bought them nice things he could get head for desert.

This is what I explained as I gave my own answer in the thread. I told them that most men believe that all women suck dick because the vast majority do, they just don't want to admit it. You can just about imagine the brigade of appalled responses I got from the women when I said this.

I politely explained to them what a lot of their parents had refused. I told them that if they reserved sex, of any kind, especially oral for someone special then they wouldn't have to be ashamed to admit it. As long as it's with two consenting adults who care about each other and proper safety measures were practiced then there was no need to hide behind lies. It only becomes something filthy and something to be ashamed of when you are sucking off every dick in a ten mile radius. Or if you have fell for the okie doke that I spoke about in volume one of **The Love Den Diaries – From Dating Disaster To Dating Master**, meaning you went for the old "we are just kicking it , let's have casual sex with no title" AKA friends with benefits. Now you feel bad because you have given up once again something that should be reserved for someone special to a random fling. Sounds pretty silly right? Would you admit to it?

Another reason some women cringe at the thought of giving head is the end result. The fact that they know he might possibly blow a load of semen in their mouth repulses them to no end. Some women are under the impression that cum is something nasty and that they may even get sick if they ingest it. Others find the whole act of swallowing offensive and degrading. So with that being said let's explore the question: Is it REALLY ok to swallow?

Semen, or cum, is actually made up of 90 percent seminal fluids including fructose (sugar) and proteins; sperm accounts for only about one percent of its total volume and the rest is made up of trace minerals and nutrients. And rest assured ladies semen is not fattening. It only contains about 12 to 15 calories per serving. This be would equivalent to one egg white.

Taking semen into the mouth is safe, as is swallowing semen, unless the semen has a sexually transmitted infection in it, in which case you need to avoid any type of sexual contact altogether. Using the proper precautionary measures will help lessen the chances of spreading infection and disease. This can be achieved by either using a latex condom (preferably flavored). I cannot scream this enough. PLEASE do not take chances with your health or life for that matter by having unprotected sex of any kind.

Unprotected oral sex can put both giver and receiver at risk of sexually transmitted diseases such as; Gonorrhea, Hepatitis B, Herpes, Human Papilloma Virus (HPV), Syphilis, and, rarely, Chlamydia and HIV. If the guy has wounds on his genitals, or if the giving partner has wounds or open sores on or in his or her mouth, or bleeding gums, this poses an increased risk of STD transmission.

Also remember that brushing the teeth, flossing, undergoing dental work, or eating crunchy foods such as potato chips relatively soon before or after giving head can also increase the risk of transmission, because all of these activities can cause small scratches in the lining of the mouth.

Some women say that the taste of cum is unpleasant, bitter, salty, or even acidic. However there are specific things a man can do which will improve the taste. Some women swallow semen and actually enjoy it, it's because their male partners have probably been considerate enough to improve the taste of their semen by following some of the tips given by Mans Health Magazine Online:

Since semen is excreted by the body, male semen taste and smell would most likely be affected by what you eat and drink. So, are there foods that affect the taste of semen and are actually able to change the way it tastes? What's the best diet for improving semen taste?

For one, you should start living a clean and healthy lifestyle. Cut down and even eliminate alcohol, drugs and nicotine. Avoid junk foods and instead have lots of fruits and greens in your diet. Drink plenty of water.

Drinking fruit juices from pineapple, citrus, and cranberry is also known to make semen taste sweeter. Throw in melon, mango, apple, or grape, and other fruits that are high in sugar. Likewise, vegetables like parsley and celery are recommended.

There are also some foods that you should steer clear of. Fish and red meat produce a bitter, fishy male semen taste because of their alkaline content. Chemically-processed alcohol can also make your semen taste bitter. Instead, try naturally fermented drinks for a change. Garlic and onion are likely to produce strong odors since they are high in sulfur; so avoid these as well.

Chapter 2 -The Fellatio Frame Of Mind

You've heard it said a million times, attitude is everything. This goes for everything that you do in life, and giving head no different. Believe it or not getting yourself in the right frame of mind outside of the bedroom will affect your performance inside the bedroom. One of the first things you can do to improve your sex life is to change your attitude towards giving oral sex.

Whether you are a woman who really doesn't mind going down on her man but rather just need a few tips and techniques to help you step your game up, or if you are someone who is shy and apprehensive about the whole idea, you are reading the right book. In this chapter you will learn how to mentally and physically prepare to do the deed.

One of the best pieces of advice that I can give to a man or a woman in the sex department is to get acquainted with each other's bodies as well as your own. Oral sex should not be reserved only for when you are having vaginal sex. You need to open your mind to exploring every inch of your lover's body. This a guaranteed way of knowing what makes their spine tingle and their eyes roll back.

If it's been ages since you have given your man a REAL blow job he will more than welcome your "practice sessions." These sessions should not be done during a time when you are feeling rushed or super tired.

Part of the physical and mental preparation for this session is to take a nice hot shower or bath and relax. Gather any needed "props", if you prefer, some soft music, and a glass of wine wouldn't hurt either.

You guys need to think of this not as a night of romance with expectations of back breaking sex. These sessions are your "classes." You need to express to your guy that you are willing to please him and that you want to get to know what turns him on WITHOUT the pressure of him having to perform. For some men this will be a great relief if they have never ejaculated from receiving oral sex. It gives him a chance in a non-expectation environment to not only receive pleasure; but to teach you what he likes as well.

I honestly believe if people approached sex with a more laid back attitude and a bit of humor it would make both parties feel more at ease. Communication is key in every element of your relationship and sex should not be an exception.

Another thing you need to do is make YOURSELF feel sexy. That means even though you may be tired from working, doing chores around the house, and taking care of the kids you need to still take time out for yourself.

Quite often we get in a rut and tend to take care of everything else and everyone else except ourselves. Sometimes that means letting your weight get out of hand, your hair hasn't been styled in ages and you are sporting chipped up polish on your finger nails and toe nails.

You might be asking yourself; what do these things have to do with me giving good head. What does feeling sexy have to do with my performance? It's quite simple. When you feel good about yourself you will be more confident. That means if you need to lose those extra few pounds so that you don't have to hide behind mounds of clothing every time you go to bed then so be it.

There are many women who refuse to let their man actually see their body when having sex. They either come to bed dressed like they are going hiking or they insist on keeping the lights out. This chapter is not about putting anyone down for their weight, but rather getting you to understand that you need to feel comfortable in your own skin no matter what your size.

The weight was just one example of how you can feel self-conscious in the bedroom. As I stated before it could be hair, nails, lack of energy, etc... The point I'm trying to make is men love it when a woman, no matter what she looks like, feels and shows that she is sexy and confident within herself. This will make for better sex because you will more than likely be less inhibited in between the sheets. And who wouldn't love that!

Some women need to get themselves in the mood beforehand. They need to first be turned on themselves before they can turn their lover on. This means that you may need to watch a skin flick, curl up with an erotic novel, masturbate or all of the above. The whole idea is you want to feel sexy, hot, desirable, and eager to please going into the act. Instead of stressed tired, bored, and feeling blah all the way around.

Mental preparation is not only essential for you but for your guy as well. We know very well that most men will willingly accept a blow job with no questions asked, at the drop of a hat. That's all fine and dandy, but how much better would it be if you spent a little time throughout your day making him feel wanted?

Contrary to belief women aren't the only ones who want and NEED to feel desired. For that reason you should start stroking and teasing him mentally long before you actually plan on going down on him. If you see each other in the morning before you leave for work try coming up behind him and grabbing his package while he has his morning wood. Whisper in his ear what you plan to do with it later on that evening/night. BEWARE: This one may lead to him wanting you at that very moment, which is fine as long as time permits. You could also send him naughty text messages throughout the day telling him how bad you want him, or how you've been waiting to taste him all day. If you get a chance when you slip away to lunch get something to suck on like a lollipop or a piece of candy, call him up and let him hear you actually sucking it. Tell him you are pretending that it's him. After all this mental masturbation beforehand he will be ready to shoot off like a bottle rocket when you finally see each other!

The very fact that you are reading this book says that you want to step your head game up. However for anything to work you MUST first try it. You can't expect to spice up your sex life without putting in the necessary work. If at any time you feel like it's too much work or your man is not worth it, due to the fact that you two have issues outside the bedroom, or he's a lazy lover, then you need to reevaluate what the relationship means to you and what you are getting from it. In my opinion if they aren't worthy of the work, then they are not worthy of the relationship.

Chapter 3 - Do I Really Have to Return The Favor?

I'm gonna start this chapter out by saying that you know you are dead ass wrong for even asking that question. If you have ever had a sexual relationship with someone who was a selfish lover then you know all too well how frustrating it can be watching the other person get off over and over while you lay there wondering what the hell is going on.

For those of you who don't what a selfish lover is, it's someone who only thinks of themselves when it comes to sex. Not surprisingly this trait usually carries over to other parts of the relationship as well. The selfish lover will make sure they "get theirs" meaning they are going to get off at any cost. If you don't "get yours" oh well, it's just too bad.

This type of lover will want you to go down

on them but refuse to return the favor. Or they will outright refuse sex altogether just because THEY aren't in the mood. Some will even go as far as using sex as a weapon to punish if they feel like their partner has wronged them. And just as sex is used as a weapon, oral sex runs a close second.

There are people who will in fact go down on their lover, but only a special occasion, if they want something, or if they need to use it as part of a makeup session after a fight. You guessed it. It's straight up manipulation and control for some. For others it's a matter of them just being a spoiled brat and use to getting their own way. Their lover's pleas for them to satisfy them go ignored until someone either cheats, calls it quits, or continues on but remains bitter.

For many years women have used sex as a way of getting whatever they want from a man, even if this meant costing them their marriage. It's no wonder the men are turning the tables when it comes to withholding. One of our shows on Chattin with Candace and Midnite titled: My Man Is Rationing The Dick remains our number one most downloaded show.

I must put a disclaimer out there now that states: withholding has been typically done by women when it comes to sex, however there are passive aggressive men who use the "I have a headache" excuse more than women for something as simple as they were angry because they didn't want to make the trip to the mall.

And yes ladies I know many of you complain that YOU are the ones not receiving oral pleasure. Several of you have said that you have stopped taking care of your man in that department because as I started before he was a selfish lover or he didn't know what he was doing when he got down there. I can't express this enough, PLEASE take the time to learn what YOUR lover likes in the bedroom.

This goes for men and women alike. The moves that made your ex husband/wife scream to the rooftop may barely get a moan from your current lover. And as I stated in Chapter three, if your partner outright refuses to try and make the necessary changes to improve your sex life you might want to consider counseling if you are married or moving on if you are not.

Hopefully reading this chapter will give you some insight into why it is ABSOLUTELY necessary to return the favor. This doesn't mean that every time you have sex you should be required to suck him off, just as he shouldn't be required to slurp you up. However letting your lover lick you into a coma from multiple orgasms and not expecting him to want the same pleasure in return is a bit unrealistic and need I say it again selfish.

And speaking of slurping let's talk about the swallowing double standard. I know numerous women who detest even being asked to suck dick. At least that's what they say in public. God forbid a man wants them to swallow. However these same women will drown a man in her love juices. Not to mention cutting off his breath as she's nearing orgasm from her thighs locked on his head like a vice grip.

So what's the deal? Why is there a double standard when it comes to giving head versus eating pussy? Ladies why do you require your man to slurp you up like a big gulp from 7 11 but shriek in disgust if he asks you to do the same? You really need to think about the fact that you don't want semen anywhere near you while you are drowning him in your sea of love liquids or strangling him with your thighs in a death grip when you cum. And we won't even go there with you squirters. You damn near put his eye out last time you made love and you still have the nerve to complain.

Ok so let's size it up.

The women have to deal with the gag reflex, maybe a little pube hair in the mouth, a little prejack fluid in the beginning, moderate amount of bitter fluid, but not till the very end, and worst case scenario some funky balls, in which case you should be backing off anyway.

For the men: Instant and steady flow of juices. (usually an acquired taste), pube hairs if she hasn't shaved, possible strangulation from locking thighs, possible smothering if she's sitting on her man's face and loses balance, chance of smelly tuna. Again I say keep it moving. Unlike with us ladies, swallowing sperm is actually the fastest way of getting rid of it without tasting it. That's not the case for the guys, they are tasting you the entire time.

Swallowing is not a requirement for every man and for those that like it, it's usually not a requirement every time. Most men who receive head from their lady and she refuses to swallow are fine with her spitting as long as he gets that nut (at least that's what they tell you).

However even with that being said let's not get it twisted. Swallowing is like the icing on the cake, it's the ying to his yang, it's what peanut butter is to jelly, and a cigarette is to a smoker after good sex or a good meal. In other words it's the shit! And quite frankly you would be surprised to find out how many men REALLY want their woman to swallow their seed. But they refuse ask because it was a chore just getting you to go down in the first place.

Keep in mind this book is NOT about convincing you to swallow semen, but rather to teach you that it's ok if you choose to do so, and how much enjoyment your man will get from you doing it. The book is also a guide to understanding that it's ok to give a blow job and not feel ashamed, or feel uneasy every time the subject comes up in a conversation.

Also in the words of one of my prior forum members who happens to be a guy:

"Once a woman's juices start flowing, any man that's eating it right will be swallowing the entire time he's down there... on the other hand many women tend to get queasy or offended even at the thought of swallowing. I had an ex that literally stopped every minute or so to spit out anything she might have gotten in her mouth... needless to say that was a huge turn off. Swallowing isn't a requirement of mine all the time, but I hate when it's getting good and she stops to go spit just because I came, I'm sorry please swallow and keep going just like you would want me to do after you cum."

Can you see where the problem is here ladies? Can you understand how stopping to spit or wiping your mouth every few minutes can be a straight up passion killer? If your man was to treat your juices in this manner or appear to be appalled at the very thought of putting his mouth on you, your feelings would surely be hurt.

In another forum where men were asked why

they loved a woman to swallow, these were their answers:

"For me personally, I find it a huge turn-off if the girl spits after I've cum in her mouth. For her to accept it, and then swallow it makes the whole procedure seamless and more natural. If she pretends to swallow it, then goes to the bathroom later and discreetly gets rid of it, that's OK, too."

"Because it is incredibly erotic, it is the grand finale of the act of the blow job. It doesn't feel properly complete unless the cum slides down your throat. It indicates that you are enjoying yourself as well and that he is providing you sustenance."

"Most of us don't care, definitely not a deal breaker, but there's something about a woman taking you "all in" that is very exciting, not sure how to explain it."

"There's something sexier about a girl who isn't grossed out by it."

"The one blow job I've had where the woman actually swallowed was the most amazing experience of my life. As I nutted she continued sucking and it was the most intense orgasm I've ever had. The fact that she swallowed it just multiplied my level of arousal."

Bottom line: Swallowing is a huge turn on for some men, others could care less as long as they get off. However the choice is entirely up to the woman. Just remember if you choose not to swallow please don't make it seem as though you are totally grossed out (even if you are). This is a huge turn off for men. And if you do decide to swallow just know that the gesture will be well received.

Chapter 4 - Become A Dick Sucking Diva

In this chapter you will learn all the tricks of the trade. For the less experienced divas the information provided will help you to give Karrine Steffans a run for her money. For the more seasoned ladies I'm positive there will be some tips that will help you step your game up as well.

Before we dig in I would like to share some

of the responses from the men when asked in a sex forum "What makes a blow job great?"

"For her to take her time....savor it.....enjoy it for herself and pretend mankind existence depends on her performance lol. Plus be creative.... if she just doing it because....it takes the fun out of it!"

"Passion, you just got to love doing it."

"Mechanically, you got to play with the nuts and the taint. Use your hand and mouth to switch it up so you don't get tired. Make a tight coochie with your tongue and the top of your mouth so it can't choke you. And be a little rough with it."

"If you really want to impress him. Suck until he nuts and then suck until he gets hard again. Then fuck him. Don't do this if you think he has stalking tendencies."

"Lick the shaft and stroke/lick the balls, and then mix it up. Keep it interesting, if you find a rhythm he likes, don't stop. NO TEETH!"

"What I don't want is an expert... I know that

sounds completely odd but the biggest turn off to me is a blow job expert. I could care less how many dicks you have sucked and how great you believe you are at it... you're dealing with mine now take your cues from me. In the beginning sure go ahead and do your thing, after all I don't know what to expect.... but there will be a time where I start to give some pointers... don't ignore them and do not convince yourself that you know what's best for me... if you were doing what I liked I'd just lay back/sit there/stand there and enjoy it. If I move your head around, don't be offended just go with it... If I pull it out your mouth and hold the head... that just means the rest of the shaft and the balls want some attention too. If I stop you and start fucking your face, just hold still I'm enjoying it This doesn't mean that I'm opposed to kicking back and letting her do her thing.... who knows she might bring something new to the table."

"I prefer a woman to swallow if the moment requires it... meaning if you have me in that right spot don't stop to go spit or anything like that it just ruins the vibe, just swallow and keep going. It's not over for me just because I ejaculated... I'd like to enjoy my orgasm if you may, just like a woman wants to enjoy hers... keep going until I stop quivering."

"Ice/peppermint/Altoids/warm tea/Listerine all these aid in making a great blow job. Truly what makes a great blow job is the interest and attention into the act. If you make it seem like you are really into it, like you truly are enjoying giving as you want us to be pleasured, that's makes a great blow job. Don't make it seem like you have other things you could be doing besides this. We are not detached from our penis. Similar to you are not detached from your vagina. The luxury you have is that there are so many options to make it pleasurable for you. If you want him fresh, say "I so enjoy tasting you fresh out the shower." Say this and see how many baths he will take. What guy doesn't like visual acts? If you like icecream grab some and some nice smooth caramel and go to town. Take a small scoop in your mouth. Drizzle some caramel syrup on the dick and go to work. Do you like the taste of peppermint? Then take a candy cane and place it against the penis sucking both at the same time. All of this aids in helping you and making it pleasurable for him."

"Yes some warm peppermint or green tea. Held in the mouth and then slowly go down on him. There is no better sensation than the feeling of the warmth from the tea. It can't be hot mind you. Slightly warm and it's absolutely great, especially if it has a minty sensation. To really enhance the experience, drop a peppermint in the tea. Or take an Altoid and then drink the tea, i you want him to run not climb, but run up a wall!"

Get the point ladies? The guys want you into it!

Now it's time to move on to the good stuff. Let's get to the tips!

1. **Get Comfortable:** One of the worst things you can do when giving your man a blow job is to just jump right in only to later realize that your neck, head or body is in an awkward position. Or your knees are killing you from kneeling on hardwood or tile.

   If your guy likes receiving head with you on your knees you need to make sure that a pillow is always close by. You might even try keeping one slipped under the edge of the bed or tucked away in the hall closet for that unexpected romp on the living room floor. Also keep in mind that positioning yourself correctly when he's lying back will help you to avoid neck strain. One of the most comfortable positions for sucking him off is to have him lie flat on his back with you between his legs rather than trying to approach from the side. Always remember ladies, just because you are pleasing him doesn't mean it should be uncomfortable for you.

2. **Lick It Like A Lollipop:** How many licks does it take to get to the center of a tootsie pop? If you are old enough to remember that commercial and candy you surely remember licking and sucking till you just about had lockjaw trying to get to the center. Well that's your goal when sucking his dick. We want what's in the center to (cum) forth.

    If you are just starting to do the deed you will want to use just enough pressure to tease him mercilessly. If this is done correctly he will be on the brink of explosion by the time the real sucking starts. Start at the base of his penis and work your way to the tip using your lips to gently kiss every inch of his dick. Then use your tongue to lick the shaft.

Make sure you pay special attention the helmet (tip) switching from gently flicking your tongue across it to giving it a little suck and sometimes a slight nibble. BE CAREFUL WITH THOSE TEETH! Keep your eyes and ears open for moans and facial expressions that let you know he's enjoying what you are doing. Some men are super sensitive when it comes to the head of their penis. This means he may want you to back off a bit and then work your way back to it. It may also means for some guys teeth are out of the question PERIOD.

Also be sure to deliberately let him feel your warm breath caressing him during the process. This will make for a better sensation rather than just stroking him with a stiff dry tongue.

3. **Warning: Slippery When Wet:** Speaking of a dry tongue this is something you will want to be aware of. When getting him off orally you want your mouth to mimic a pussy as close as possible. This means the wetter the better. How would you feel if he went down on you with a tongue feeling like sandpaper? You would be pissed because it's not a good feeling.

   To combat the issue of dry mouth IE you running out of spit, try keeping a beverage or a few of your favorite flavored lubricants close at hand..

4. **Make It Rough, Make It Smooth:** Try experimenting with different textures. Keep in mind this can start with your tongue. Due to the raised taste buds the front will feel a bit rougher than the back. Try switching back and forth between the two for a unique sensation.

   You could also try wearing a pair of satin gloves and stroking him with both hands. Many men love the feel of silky fabric against their skin. This is why most lingerie is designed with that purpose in mind. Some men even enjoy the feeling of a nubby fabric that creates more friction such as a soft corduroy or velvet. Try wrapping your hand in one of these materials before stroking his shaft.

5. **Don't Fake it!:** If you really don't want to give your man a blow job it WILL SHOW! One of the biggest complaints that most men have when it comes to receiving oral sex is that fact that his lady is not into it. Imagine a guy going down on you and he squirmed the entire time he was down there. What if he made facial express that showed he didn't like what he tasted or smelled; or if he acted like the whole act of licking the kitty completely grossed him out? This would not leave you feeling very desirable.

    And I have news for you ladies; don't think that just because you are doing a lousy job that he will stop wanting oral sex. He may have just gotten to the point to where he doesn't ask YOU for it, but that doesn't mean he still doesn't crave it. Men are no different than women in this area, in the fact they want to feel wanted and desired just like you do.

6. **Get Me Bodied!:** Rub his dick on your body. Nothing turns a man on more than feeling a nice pair of tits wrapped around his boner. If your guy is into titty fucking you can lie on your back and give him both the pleasure of sucking him off while he slides his penis between your breasts.

If he's into feet you could start by teasing him with your toes stroking his shaft. You can also assume the girl on top position and use tip of his dick to caress the insides of your thighs, finally letting it touch Miss Kitty. DO NOT let it slide in! You only want him to feel how warm and wet you are for him, and then it's back to giving head. The whole idea is to tease and arouse.

7. **The Toe Curlers:** Just like experimenting with different textures

can heighten arousal, so can the sensations of, warmth, cold, slippery, tingly, etc.

The urban dictionary describes a method of sucking dick that gives your man the feeling of a velvet tongue. This is where a little preparation is needed. You will make yourself a cup of tea (not too hot) then add a spoon of honey to your mouth. After taking a sip of the tea proceed to suck him off. The heat from the tea and your mouth will melt the honey giving him the sensation of "velvet." Also the honey gives you a nice flavor to taste while doing the deed.

Another sensation would be the coolness of your mouth after sucking on a peppermint or swishing your mouth with mouthwash beforehand. The tingling is a surefire way to get his temperature rising! Be sure to use something minty! Do not use Listerine or anything cinnamon. If it burns your mouth what do you think it will do to his genitals?

Keep in mind that a cool/cold mouth can feel just as good on him as a warm one. Try sucking on ice chips at the same time you are sucking him just be sure that there are no sharp edges. If that's too intense for him try periodically taking sips of a cool beverage.

8. **Lick The Line:** This is the skin region between the anus and the scrotum. You know that little line of skin under his balls ladies? This line connects the balls to the anus called the perineum. The slang terms that are commonly used for this area of the human body, are most commonly gooch, taint, the ABC or Ass Ball Connection.

   This patch of skin is packed with nerve endings. It is a very high erogenous zone. Licking or gently sucking this area will drive him crazy and when he feels the warmth and moisture from your soft wet lips coupled with the heat from your breath. His hair will be standing on edge in no time!

9. **Deep Throat When Swallowing:** This

tip is for those of you ladies who don't mind giving head but despise the taste of semen. Deep throating your guy when he is near climax and let the cum slid down into the throat by itself. Ask your guy to alert you when he is about to cum. He can either verbalize it or maybe a tap on your head or shoulder. Then move his penis as far back in your mouth as possible.

You will lessen your chances of tasting most of the fluid, more so than having him in the front of your mouth. This is because there are no taste buds on the back of the tongue Once you get this technique down you can let his cum hit the back of your throat totally bypassing the tongue altogether. Before you know it, all the cum is inside you and you've barely tasted a thing.

10. **Sweeten The Load:** This is another one for the ladies who hate the taste of cum. Keep in mind that certain foods will contribute to how his load tastes. Some foods can even improve the taste somewhat. Citrus, especially, is good for

this. Drinking a lot of juice (pineapple seems to work best) should affect the taste enough to make it bearable.

11. **Suck Him Hard And Swallow Him Fast:** Once a guy starts to spew, one of the biggest mistakes that most women make is letting his load fill your mouth. If you have followed the previous tips for having him at the back of your throat, your battle is halfway over. You need to then be sure to swallow fast. Try your best to take it down as he shoots it out. Once again this is a move that will require practice but if you don't like the taste of semen, this will help get it down faster.

12. **Hey Kool Aid!:** Remember how much you loved Kool Aid as kid? Well now is the perfect opportunity to bring back those old memories of eating the sweetened kind straight out of the pack (yes kids really did sneak and do this). Grab your favorite flavor of presweetened Kool Aid and give his dick a dunk! As you suck him clean you kill two birds with one stone by not only

giving him pleasure, but by making it fun and flavorful for yourself as well!

13. **Control The Sharp Shooter:** Some men blow their load with force, especially if he's really turned on. The fact that he is exploding like fireworks on the fourth of July stimulates the gag reflex in some women even if they are swallowing as fast as they can. This can be avoided by controlling his flow of semen by either pulling back a bit (yes you will taste it then), or directing the load to the side of your mouth then swallowing in one big gulp.

14. **Let's Play Ball!:** The tip and the shaft of his dick are not the only parts that want attention. The next time you go down on your man be sure to handle his balls as well, preferably simultaneously while sucking him off. Some men like a bit of a rough handling when it comes to their sac. However you MUST pay attention to his reactions as well as start off gently and increase pressure gradually based on his reaction. And remember one wrong move could cause

him discomfort. Each guy is different so be sure to pick up on his cues so that you know when you are handing them just right.

15. **Time For Tea:** Tea bagging that is, don't be afraid to work your way down with your mouth and flick your tongue across his scrotum. If you are lying on your back he may want to dip those balls in your mouth, in and out. Hence the name tea bagging because it resembles a tea bag being dipped in and out of a cup. Not only do you want to lick his balls you want to tease him to the point of orgasmic orbit by gently taking them in your mouth and rolling them around with your tongue. You can also wrap your lips around one at a time and suck away!

16. **The Jaw Breaker:** Use your hands as well as your mouth. Most men prefer to have their dick stroked simultaneously while you suck them off. You can alternate playing with their balls as well. This will take some of the work away from your jaws as they tire and give

them a break, hence the title jawbreaker.

17. **Suck Hard On The Come Up:** This is the technique of sucking him harder on the upstroke and softer on the down stroke. If you learn to master this it will also help save your jaws some of the work while making him squirm with delight.

18. **I've Got My Eye On You:** This move tends to weird some guys out so you will have to feel him out on this one. Try looking at him while you are going down on him. Don't make it a blank serial killer, I'm gonna bite your dick off stare, but more like a demure, coy, sexy look, as though you were saying: "I'm so happy to be pleasing you." For some men this is an extreme turn on seeing his lady in a vulnerable position and looking so intent on satisfying his every need.

19. **Talk Dirty:** This is a hit with most guys, they love nothing more than to hear you talk raunchy in the bedroom, especially if it's the complete opposite of

the real you in everyday life. Start by whispering in his ear as you work your way down his body with kisses. Tell him how bad you want to taste him. Once you finally arrive at your destination be sure to tell him how good his dick tastes. This is like a dream come true for most men. Not only because you have gone down on him, but to see that you are actually enjoying doing it.

20. **Worship The Dick:** I don't mean that literally. It just means that it's imperative that you LOOK like you are enjoying pleasing him. If you combine the act of actually wanting to give him oral pleasure along with the talking dirty tips that I gave above you will have one happy guy on your hands. As I previously stated, one of the biggest complaints among men when they receive head is the fact that his lady looks so disinterested while preforming it, and even seems to look relieved when it's over.

21. **Let Him Face Fuck You:** This is the

method of letting HIM guide your head as you suck. He will usually hold the back of your head or depending on how freaky you guys are he can pull your hair as he fucks away at your face.

22. **Turn That Dick Into A Banana Split!:** Gather all the topping for a banana split except the banana. His dick will serve that purpose. Cover those nuts with some real nuts and Cool Whip. And a little chocolate syrup, a few fruit toppings and devour him up!

23. **Let The World See:** Please be careful with this one. We don't want you to go to jail for indecent exposure while trying to play out a voyeurism fantasy. Depending on how daring you are you can suck him off while sitting in the back of a dark theater, the drive in movie, in a parked car in a wooded area, etc... Let your imagination run wild. The fun behind this technique is the thrill of getting caught while not actually doing so. The experience can be quite an adrenalin rush of mind blowing sex.

24. **Play Dress Up:** Fantasy role play is always a welcome addition in the bedroom. Try wearing a wig in a different hair color than your own hair. If you normally don't wear lipstick invest in a bright red shade just for going down on him .This will make for a nice visual as you lick and tease his body into another dimension. Don't forget to throw on a nice pair of stilettos along with some sexy black stockings. With an outfit like this he will definitely want to finish up by laying the pipe to your sexy ass!

25: **The Vacuum Effect:** Try sucking on his member creating a vacuum-like tightness   and pressure. Don't be afraid to suck hard, most guys enjoy that strong sensation. Suck on the head, or take the whole cock in your mouth and maintain the suction the entire time you slide it in and out of your mouth.

25. **Prolong His Pleasure:** Ask your guy to alert you when he feels the sensation of orgasm approaching, lightly tug downward on his testicles (they tend to

rise closer to the body when he's near orgasm) can delay ejaculation. Remember to gently tug; don't yank.

26. **Different Stokes:** The standard up and down stroke can be effective when sucking him off or giving him a hand job, but it can also get boring and quickly lead to over-stimulation. Experiment with different kinds of strokes, alternating between your hands and your mouth. Use a twisting motion while moving up and down; roll his dick between your palms, alternate short strokes at the base of his cock with longer strokes at the tip. Or you could start with short strokes at the tip and gradually make them longer at the base. Instead of moving up and down, try only stroking up and away from the body.

27.: **Make It A Surprise:** Keep him guessing what sensation is going to come next by blindfolding him. Or if he's up for it you can hand cuff him as well. Many men love the idea of taking on a submissive role when it comes to sex.

Since this technique will be done on someone who trusts you, be sure not to break that trust. That means no sharp contrasts between hot/cold smooth/rough. Be sure gradually ease into each move preferably touching an area like his inner thigh or belly first if you are using something like ice or a feather to tickle. This way he will still get surprise of the new sensation but it will put him at ease knowing what's about to come near his package.

Also keep in mind that anytime there is bondage or blindfolds involved the person on the receiving end needs "safe" words to use. These words set boundaries by signaling their partner to ease up or stop what they are doing altogether. Wiki describes safe words as follows: A safe word needs to be something one can remember and call to mind when things are either not going as planned or have crossed a threshold one cannot handle. The most commonly used form of safe words are: green, yellow, and red. Red meaning to stop and there would be no further play. Yellow being, this is getting too intense. Green meaning that everything is okay. It's all about trust.

28.: **Chest Release:** For the times when you don't plan on swallowing let him shoot his load on your tits. Use your hands to squeeze them around his dick as he slides in and out between them.

29.: **Get Your Nibble On:** Nibble your way up the side of his dick as if it were corn on the cob, taking the skin lightly between your lips or teeth and tugging gently. Believe it or not, it is possible to please him in this manner without inducing pain. Normally penises and teeth don't like each other, but if done correctly this move can drive him to the point of no return!

30.: **Pop his cork:** Turn his dick into a bubbling sensation by taking a swig of champagne and holding it in your mouth while sucking him off. If you pair it with an Altoids mint it will create a fizzing, bubbly eruption in your mouth that's bound to send him into orbit!

31. **Lights, Camera, Action!:** This is another one that depends on trust. Depending on how adventurous you are you can let your guy star in his very own skin flick. You can either let him hold the camera or position it so it catches all the steamy details. This little flick will make for some great foreplay or solo action later on.

32. **Gumming The Dick**: Yeah that's right I said it! For all you seniors out there who are still trying to get their groove on, pop out those dentures and go to work! This move can actually be done by anyone who is missing teeth. Hey don't knock it till you've tried it!

33.: **Wow Him With Water:** Consider investing in a removable adjustable shower head if you haven't done so already. The next time he takes a shower join him. Position yourself on your knees in front of him. You will need a mat or bath pillow for your comfort. Have him get the water to just the right temperature then hold his dick and suck it with one hand while the other hand uses the spray nozzle to stimulate his balls. Some men are very sensitive in this area so be sure to adjust the water pressure to his comfort level. While you are down there licking and teasing spray back and forth across balls back toward his anus. As the pleasure and intensity increases so can the pressure of the water.

34. **Smoke It Like A Bong:** I'm not advocating smoking weed but ahem just in case you do, you can try this move. Before you go down on him take a hit off of a joint/blunt. Then proceed to take his cock in your mouth along with the smoke. The warm heat from the smoke will give him a tantalizing sensation. As you slide up and down on the dick blow the smoke out of your nose. Repeat this action till he blows his load.

35. **Coax The Turtle Out Of Its Shell:** Is your man working with an uncircumcised dick? We haven't forgotten about him. Hold on to the

shaft of his penis and tease the tip of the head by sticking your tongue in the foreskin. Do this until the head surfaces from him becoming erect. Just like a turtle peeking out of his shell. Keep in mind that because it's protected by the foreskin, the head is really sensitive, and too much direct stimulation can feel uncomfortable.

Also make sure you involve the foreskin in the blow job process. Do not just push it aside like it's in the way. The foreskin has a ton nerve endings in it as well so be sure to let your tongue go to work!

36. **Skittle Dick:** This is one you will really want to be careful with so you don't choke. Take a handful of Skittles into your mouth then take his dick in your mouth along with the Skittles. As you suck up and down, roll them around in your mouth to create a massaging sensation. This can get pretty messy from all the juicy goodness from the candy creating the extra saliva you need to keep him lubed up as well as sending

him over the rainbow.

37. **Morning Glory:** What man wouldn't appreciate his lady waking him with some good head? You can either gown down on him while he's sleep, before he wakes up in the morning. Or pull a sneak attack in the middle of the night.

38. **Fizzy pop:** Oldie but goodie. Stop by the candy store and pick up some pop rock candy. Place a handful in your mouth and suck his dick while the rocks explode. Take extra precaution not to choke while doing this.

39. **Give Him A Throat Massage:** Once you learn to master the deep throat technique, contract your throat muscles while he's inside your mouth, massaging the head of his dick. Giving him a sensation he won't soon forget.

40. **Stay Alert:** Pay attention to your partner's responses. Don't get so caught up into what you're doing that you ignore how he's responding. As you change rhythms, methods, or where

you're touching, look for little signals of his pleasure and give him more of whatever he seems to be enjoying the most!

41. **Juice Him Up!:** Hollow out the center of a large orange and slide it over his penis. Be sure to slide it all the way through. We don't want any of that juice getting in his pee hole because it may burn. As you lick and suck his shaft and balls, squeeze the orange and let the juice drip down. Proceed to lap up all the juicy goodness!

42. **Go Numb:** Use an anesthetic spray like Chloraseptic to spray the back of your throat just before giving head. This will lessen the gag reflex when you start deep throating him. Please be aware that some men are very sensitive to any kind of numbing agent and doing so will cause the head their dick to go numb as well, prolonging their orgasm. This is fine if you are dealing with a guy who prematurely ejaculates. However if you're not you could be sucking all night. In which case you will need to

drink something after the numbing takes effect on your throat to wash away any direct reside that could cause this issue.

43. **Flick The Frenulum:** Place your mouth over the top of the dick and start flicking his frenulum in a quick motion with your stiff tongue. This is that tiny knot of flesh underneath the crown of his penis, where the head connects to the shaft. This is a super sensitive spot for a majority of men. To intensify the experience, move the circle of your thumb and forefinger up and down in a medium motion near the base of his penis. Combining this along with sucking on the head will result in an explosive orgasm.

44.: **Toss His Salad:** While going down licking his balls give him oral anal stimulation. This involves licking, flicking or inserting a stiff tongue into the anal passage. This move can also be done while he is on his knees jacking himself. You can lick his balls and anus from the back at the same time. The thrusting feels good because the area is highly sensitive and loaded with nerve endings. Your guy may like this but be too shy to tell you, so in the height of passion Do like Nike says and "Just Do It."

45.: **Press The Button:** Speaking of anal play, this is a move that will require you to proceed with caution. This may scare your guy and kill the whole mood. So you may want to suggest this one beforehand to get his feedback. However if he's comfortable with it, while going down on him use the tip of your finger to press on his anus. Do not insert your finger. Simply press and massage the area hard enough to stimulate his prostate. Giving him an earth shattering orgasm!

46.: **Jump His Bone!:** Attack him when he least suspects it! When he walks in the door be aggressive! Push him against the wall and shower him with kisses. All the while you should be fondling his package. Work your way down his neck with passionate kisses. A nibble here and there won't hurt either. He'll go crazy as you release your animal lust. Drop to your knees and give him the most amazing blow job he has ever had in his life!

47.: **Let Him Dominate:** Men love feeling of dominance when it comes to receiving a blow job. Instead of always sucking him off in the bed try letting him stand with you kneeling in the floor in front of him. This can also be done while he is sitting in a chair. The whole feeling of him being in charge is a huge turn on and bound to have him reeling with pleasure.

48.: **Let Your Head Hang Low:** This move takes a little practice and it may feel uncomfortable after a prolonged period. Lay on the bed with your head hanging over the edge face up .You could also try this with your head hanging over the edge of a couch. Have your lover kneel over you and place his dick in your mouth in this position. You will notice that your tongue is flatter and you can fit more of him in your mouth. As well as your head is lined up perfectly for deep throating him with ease. For added comfort you might try having him place his hand under your head to relieve some of the strain off of your neck.

49.: **Put A Ring On It!:** A cock ring that is. They are most often used to make an erect penis harder and bigger, and to delay and heighten orgasm. Try slipping one on your man's erection before going down on him. The combination of your lips and the extra blood concentrated in his shaft from the ring, he's sure to shoot a powerful load. Note: If this is your first time using a cock ring try starting out with an adjustable one. And be sure not to tighten it to the point of cutting off circulation.

50.: **Twerk On It:** Try putting on your favorite booty shaking song and twerk your ass in front of him. This tip is actually a combination of moves. The first one being you dancing in front of him teasing him. However unlike strip tease you will not undress. You should already have on some sexy undies or skimpy shorts, preferably a slippery fabric like silk or satin.

Bounce and grind on his dick till it's hard as a rock. He can actually still have his clothes on at this point. Some men are super sensitive and the clothes will serve as a barrier to keep him from penetrating you as well as deceasing some of the sensation. We don't want him blowing his load too soon.

Once you have him fully aroused pull his dick out and proceed to give him head, alternating with a hand job. As his pleasure heightens switch back to twerking in front of him. By now he is so horny he's touching himself.

Keep in mind you are not only shaking your ass in front of him, you are grinding on his wood as well. Be sure to do this in the reverse cowgirl position so he can enjoy the view as well as grab a hold of your hips as he slides his dick up and down your ass.

Pretty soon he will be so turned on he

might even try to slip the panties to the side and hit it from the back. Don't let him penetrate you. The whole point of the dancing is to tease him to the brink of explosion. At this point you need to switch back alternating the hand job and ultimately deep throating him to finish him off.

Chapter 5 -Getting Your Girl To Go Down

You guessed it; this chapter is for the fellas. I know many of you complain that your lady will either refuse to go down on you or when she does it's basically a whack ass job because she really didn't want to do it. For many of you this has even put a strain on the relationship. You may be reading this chapter because your lady has bought this book and has shown you this section. If that is the case I would suggest that you also read Chapter Two - Yuck I Don't Want To Do That! It will give you some incite as to why your lady may be feeling a bit apprehensive when it comes to giving head.

As I have stated in previous chapters and on several of my talk shows. Sex starts well BEFORE you get in the bedroom. Granted there are women who have been conditioned to think that sucking dick is something bad because of upbringing, religious reasons, cultural beliefs, etc... However there are just as many women who refuse to do the deed simply because their man is a selfish lover, or because he has not stimulated her properly OUTSIDE of the bedroom.

Now before you get your undies in a bunch hear me out. I want to first start by saying that if you are a man that takes care of his woman in all areas of the relationship, you make her feel loved and desired as well as safe and secure then this section does not apply to you.

In fact if SHE is the one who refuses to bend in any fashion when it comes to lovemaking you need to decide what the relationship means to you. I have said it time and time again, KEEP IT MOVING if the person is not meeting your needs rather than just sticking around in a stagnate situation. Granted that doesn't mean that you are going to walk away from a long term relationship JUST because the sex is bad or because she doesn't give blow jobs. Chances are as I have said before; there are other factors that are coming into play as well. And she could just be being selfish, which would surface in other areas of the relationship as well.

You need to decide whether or not she's worth it. And no, this is NOT an excuse to cheat. If she's not satisfying you, keep it moving rather than trying to have your cake and eat it to. If she is a person that likes to play games or use sex as a weapon to try and punish I do not advocate that in any way shape or form. Now before you make this decision you need to ask yourself are YOU a game player as well? Do BOTH of you play on each other's feelings and use sex among many other things to manipulate? If that's the case then you guys have a messy situation going on and really need to do some maturing in that area.

Now that that's out of the way let's talking about those of you who KNOW that you haven't been doing everything that you should in terms of pleasing your lady. Or you know that you have been a selfish lover. You know that you haven't taken the time or the patience to know what she likes in between the sheets (and otherwise) but you expect her to please your every whim. You get your nut and roll over without giving her satisfaction a second thought. Has she ever complained to you about this? If so what did you do about it? I hate to go there but I feel I must also bring up the subject of verbal abuse. Have you called your girl out of her name and or physically abused her? Do you put her down mentally and then expect her to pretend everything is fine when it's time to get down in the bedroom? Please understand that these are not questions that I would only ask a man. I'm here to let the ladies know as well, that ANYONE, be it a man or a woman who is abusing someone in anyway is dead ass wrong.

I don't believe in withholding sex. As a matter of fact if you are in a committed relationship where two people care about each other's feelings there will be times you will have to "preform" when you don't want to. You can't always just say because I'm not in the mood or I have a funky attitude that the other person has to suffer. And I can't say it enough DO NOT use sex to manipulate. However if a person is sick or under a great deal of stress, family issues, etc... they deserve a pass.

With that being said that doesn't mean that you can call your lady a bitch in the morning and expect great head in the evening. Quite frankly in many cases where people refuse sex of any kind, men or women, it's not because they are withholding, but because they just do not want anything to do with your ass! You basically have turned them off. It's no different than your lady calling you all kinds of stupid assholes then expecting you to make passionate love to her later on. Everyone deserves to be treated with dignity and respect and when that line has been crossed you have opened up the door to much larger problems than just sex.

If any man were to ask me the secret to seduction, or the secrets to getting your lady to blowing your hair back in the sack I would say start with taking care of business OUTSIDE of the bedroom. Just as you guys love visual stimulation when it comes to sex, a woman loves mental stimulation in everyday life. If she feels like that she can count on you no matter what, and you have made her feel secure in the fact that she is the only one for you, you have the battle halfway won when it comes to getting her to please you.

The next thing would be to make sure you are doing everything in your power to please her. That means take a few extra minutes to preform foreplay, if she like to kiss then so be it. Don't always be so quick to turn her over so you can "hit it from the back" just to avoid intimacy. If you guys have been together for a while, make it a point to buy flowers for no special reason, or sneak off on a weekend get away with just the two of you. You might even pencil her in for a date night once a week.

And last but not least don't be fooled by the notion that just because we like mental stimulation that we don't like visual as well. The latter may not be as important to some women, but we do take notice when you look good and smell good, just as you do with us. Has YOUR weight gotten out of control? Does your belly rest on her head when she's trying to go down on you? This could be turning her off. What about hygiene? Do your balls smell like Blue Cheese? This could why she doesn't want to go down. Just like you don't want your lady smelling like salmon croquettes down below, you want her to smell fresh and clean. You need to extend her the same courtesy.

Also be aware of the fact that your lady may have suffered some form of sexual abuse in her lifetime. If she has ever mentioned this to you it could be why she feels apprehensive when it comes to oral sex. In any case this is a VERY delicate situation that will require much patience, caring, and understanding to work through it. You would be surprised to find out how many women have suffered this form of abuse, but have neglected to mention it to their lovers. You guys need to talk about this issue and work towards getting the counseling she may need if she hasn't done so already.

The bottom line is always keeping the lines of communication open between you two. If she is not pleasing you in the bedroom try talking to her outside of the bedroom. Ask her what are her feelings on oral sex and her reasons for not doing it. Her answers may surprise you.

Chapter 6 - Double The Pleasure Double The Fun

Ok ladies we have talked about all the different ways to please your man orally. Now we will move forward on to showing you how giving a blow job can be pleasurable for both of you. If you recall in the previous chapters I shared ways of making sure that your comfort level was not compromised just because you were going down on him. And who says that just because you are pleasing him that you can't have any fun? Exploring each other's bodies is one of the best ways to intensify your love making experience. Once again this will not work if you are dealing with a selfish lover.

One of the most common ways that couples please each other during oral sex is the 69 position. This is where both parties stimulate each other simultaneously orally. This can be done with either the man or the woman on top or side by side in the spoon position.

Another method would be to position yourself beside him as he lays back. Make sure your feet are pointing towards his head. That way he will have easy access to Miss Kitty. While you are going down on him have him fondle/finger you until he brings you to orgasm. The whole idea is for you to get yours while he's getting his. Not to mention the visual stimulation along with you getting hotter and hornier from his hands being on you is a major turn on for him.

Speaking of you getting off, why not try masturbating while he watches as you go down on him. You can use the side by side method that was listed above or you can bend over on your hands and knees with a mirror placed behind you so he can see you playing with your pussy from the back. Be sure to bounce that ass like he's hitting it from the back as well. The mere sight of him seeing you touch yourself along with your ass jiggling will get his rocks off in no time while you get your jollies as well!

If you can get past tasting his juices surely you can taste your own. Have sex with your guy as you normally would. Ask him to make sure that you get off before he orgasms. Hopefully he can last that long. If he can have him pull out just before he climaxes and finish him off orally. Or if it was feeling so amazing that he shot his load before he had a chance to pull out. Use your mouth and hands to bring him back to another erection.

Chapter 7 - Practice Makes Perfect

Just like with any masters of the trade, they practice their skill to polish their craft. This book has given you a wealth of tips to get you on your ways to becoming a blow job Samurai. Now I will share the last and final tips on how to practice doing the deed.

One of the most important things to master giving a blow job is learning how to control your gag reflex. The first thing you will want to do is relax. It is much easier to trigger this reflex when you are tensed up. This is yet another reason to calm down and take it easy when going down on him. If your mind is so dead set on how gross it will be you will send your gag reflex into overdrive.

The next thing will be to learn how to disengage your gag reflex by training it to get use to touch. Your gag reflex is triggered by a soft palate in the back of your throat designed to stop you from choking. By gradually getting your soft palette use to being touched, you can minimize the gag reflex, or perhaps even get rid of it completely. This is one of the methods used by sword swallowers.

You can use your toothbrush for this exercise. What you want to do is slowly work it to the back of your mouth till you stimulate this reflex. Once it starts, relax and let it happen. Yes it will be unpleasant, but the whole idea is to "tickle" that area every day for about 10 seconds.

Open your mouth, stick your tongue out, and use the toothbrush to find exactly where your gag reflex is. You'll know when you've hit it because, well, you'll start gagging. Now, take your toothbrush and gently scrub that area for ten seconds, or as long as you can before you feel like you are about to vomit. Repeat this step at least once a day. As you become more comfortable start brushing further down the back of your tongue. You don't have to brush further than the parts of your tongue that you can see. Now you're getting the soft palate! If you don't use it, you lose it! To keep yourself in peak deep throat condition, do step three every day. After a few days you will start to notice that you gag less. Keep moving back a bit further each day.

As far as the dick sucking techniques that

have been listed; I'm sure that any man will be a more than willing candidate for participation. However if you want to surprise him with your moves you will need to practice in private.

God forbid someone sees you talking to a dildo telling it how bad you want to suck it. Yes that's right I said a dildo. You will either use a dildo or a banana for these exercises.

When you are alone you will feel less inhibited to practice "worshiping" the dick. Start by licking and sucking on the tip, and then move onward to long strokes up the sides as you curl your tongue around it. This would be a great time to try out your dirty talk. Try pretending this is your man's dick. Talk to him. Tell him what you want to do with his dick and how bad you want to suck it. Get use to the feel of it in your hands. Try rubbing it along your body. The whole idea is to start feeling more and more comfortable with his penis in your mouth. A banana is cool because not only does it taste good while practicing your deep throat moves. You can eat it afterward. However if your man is well endowed try grabbing yourself a dildo or cucumber in that same size, (be sure to thoroughly wash the skin first). This will help you better gauge how to wrap your lips around him and how far you will be able to take him in your mouth.

Most sex toys stores even supply ejaculating dildos. These special toys have a compartment for liquid and a hand pump to squirt it out of the dick head at the appropriate moment. This would an ideal choice for learning how to swallow. You can start with warm water but it won't be the same consistency. If you want to make it more realistic try some sugar free yogurt and add a pinch of salt. Try sucking on it, sliding it to the back of your throat then releasing a few pumps of the simulated semen. When you feel like you are getting a little seasoned, try letting it explode in your mouth at different positions. Or you could make a homemade version of this by hollowing out a cucumber and inserting a turkey baster filled with your cum substitute. It doesn't have to be a lot. Most guys only release about a tablespoon of liquid during ejaculation.

Do your jaws get tired from giving head? Get yourself some bubble gum and start chewing away. This will help strengthen your jaw muscles allowing your preform longer before running out of juice.

Always use PLENTY of saliva when going down on your man. Let it build up gradually. Not everyone is into getting a wad of spit blown onto their genitals. Practice juicing up your mouth by sucking on the dildo along with a piece of candy in your mouth. Take care not to choke as you let the wetness build.

Bonus Tips To Help You Avoid The Most Common Mistakes When Giving Head

- **Teeth:** The number one blow job mistake: letting your teeth hit his dick. I can't stress this enough ladies Ask any guy and he'll tell you over and over: nothing is worse than a blow job that is "all teeth." Teeth can nick and scrape the sensitive skin of his penis. Open your mouth wide enough that they stay away from his cock, or suck your lips in over them to cushion the rough edges.

- **Playing Beat The Clock:** Every guy likes a quickie every now and then, but unless they're in a hurry, most guys like to savor the experience of getting their dick sucked. So don't rush them. It's not a race to see how fast you can get him to cum. Take your time and he'll blow a much larger, more satisfying load.

- **Sucking Too Hard:** Even though guys like to feel what you are doing, it is possible to suck him too hard, especially the head or the helmet of the penis. It's the most sensitive part of his penis and more prone to pain and over stimulation. KEEP THE TEETH AWAY unless you are experienced in what your man likes.

- **Cracking His Nuts:** This is not some guy on the street attacking you. Use precaution anytime you are playing with his scrotum (nut sack). It's not hard to harm the family jewels. Licking, kissing, and sucking are fine. Your guy may even like a SLIGHT nibble or a little tug. Fondling them is fine too. As long as you don't squeeze them like they are in a blood pressure cuff.

- **Looking Like Dead Fish:** If a man hates when a woman lies there like a dead fish when he's fucking her, he hates getting a blow job similar to this even more. Please do not go down on him and start staring into space like you are bored to oblivion. Use your hands, body, facial expression, and voice to let him know you are into what you are doing.

- **The Light Touch:** Stroking or licking him lightly is fine when you are starting out and you are just trying to tease him. However once he is aroused and as the intensity builds you will want to make sure he "feels you." Don't be afraid to apply more pressure as you stroke/lick/suck his shaft.

- **Barfing up his seed:** If you choose not to swallow his load that's fine, but please don't attempt to swallow if you haven't mastered the gag reflex. And by all means please don't just spit it out like you totally grossed out. If you must get rid of his semen have a towel close by and discretely release it there.

- **Desert Storm:** Nothing is worse than sucking your guy off with a dry mouth. Keep it wet, very wet.

- **The Vice Grip:** Don't put his dick in a death grip. Its fine to wrap a hand around the shaft, but don't clench so hard that you cut off circulation.

Bonus Chapter - Other Erogenous Zones On Your Guy

- **His Ass:** Once again I suggest prescreening your guy for any play near the butt region. However if he's ok with it the butt cheeks are a definite hot spot for some men even though they might be ashamed to admit it. Try giving it a squeeze or fondle, if he's a freak he might want a spanking as well.The anus/rectum is a very arousing place for a lot of men. There are many nerve endings situated in the anus making it a very sensitive and pleasurable place to explore. Try using your finger or tongue to trace the outside. I DO NOT recommend inserting anything into the anus (male or female) without prior consent. In fact some men don't want you anywhere near that area, in which case you much respect his wishes.

- **The Prostate Gland (The Male G-Spot):** THIS IS NOT FOR EVERY GUY. AS I STATED BEFORE MANY MEN WILL GO POSTAL IF YOU EVEN COME NEAR THEIR ASS! THIS IS A TIP THAT MUST BE DISCUSSED BEFOREHAND. The prostate gland is the male version of the all-important and highly arousing women's G-Spot. It is located up his ass approximately 3" (8cm) inside the rectum on the front facing wall. Simply lube up your finger, slip it inside slowly and once you feel a raised bumpy area (larger in older men) motion forwards in a come to me kind of way; this should result in a deeply powerful sensation which on its own is capable of bringing a man to orgasm. Once discovered, the prostate is NEVER forgotten!

- **The Nipples:**Gently massage and kiss

the chest all over. Some men prefer firm contact and some prefer a lighter touch. Try concentrating on the nipples too but be gentle at first as it can be ticklish, applying pressure, pinching, or twisting the nipples can be highly erotic to some people but painful and uncomfortable to others. Some guys even like them sucked or gently nibbled.Other hot spots that you won't want to neglect are his lips, neck, hands, arch of his back, and feet.

To the inexperienced head giver, and the seasoned veterans alike. I hope this book has given you some tips and tricks to help to you step your head game up and keep your man happy and satisfied in the bedroom. Don't let the problems and stresses of everyday life stop you from enjoying each other to the fullest. Having great sex, oral or otherwise takes work, but it's well worth it in the end. If you have read this book to polish up your skills but you don't have any one to practice on, keep working those dildos and bananas and when you finally meet the guy whose worthy of all your tricks he will be in for the surprise of his life. To those of you who are freaks and you know it and aren't afraid to show it, more power to you. Everyone please remember to practice safe sex. And if you decide to swallow make sure you know whose seed you are ingesting. Every dick ain't gold and every pussy ain't diamonds. Don't put your mouth on anyone who can't show you that they have been tested. Better yet, go get tested together.

Until next time

Midnite Love

Cyber Slut Excerpt

"Who the hell was this calling me at this hour?" I thought to myself.

After looking at the caller ID I saw that it was Sheldon. This was when I really realized how much I liked this guy. If anyone else would have called me at this time of night knowing I had to go to work in the morning. I would have damn near cussed them out.

"Hello"

"Hey gorgeous," said Sheldon in a low husky tone.

"Hey you, what are you doing up so late?"

"Thinking about you… thinking about how bad I would love to touch you right about now. What are you wearing?"

I giggled and relaxed back onto my pillow. "If I didn't know any better I would say that someone wants some phone sex."

Sheldon laughed "Ok you busted me, but can you blame me? I'm super attracted to you

Vonne and I can't help but to wonder what it would feel like to kiss those sexy lips of yours. I'm stroking myself right now as we speak."

I didn't know whether to be repulsed or turned on. On one hand it was weird as hell having this guy call me at this hour to tell me he was jerking off thinking of me. On the other hand it had been a long time since I felt a man's hands on my body. And for some reason tonight he sounded sexy as hell.

I began tracing my nipples though my nightie till they were awakened and standing at attention. I then slid out of my panties and responded.

"I'm wearing a pink nightie without any panties" I whisper as I slowly parted my legs. "I'm attracted to you also Sheldon."

Made in the USA
Lexington, KY
18 July 2014